Fiber Intake for

Healthy Body

25 Fiber-Rich Recipes Designed to help
you Live Great

BY: SOPHIA FREEMAN

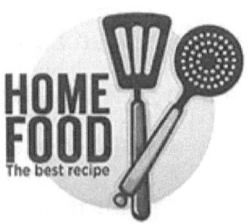

COPYRIGHTED

Liability

This publication is meant as an informational tool. The individual purchaser accepts all liability if damages occur because of following the directions or guidelines set out in this publication. The Author bears no responsibility for reparations caused by the misuse or misinterpretation of the content.

Copyright

The content of this publication is solely for entertainment purposes and is meant to be purchased by one individual. Permission is not given to any individual who copies, sells or distributes parts or the whole of this publication unless it is explicitly given by the Author in writing.

My gift to you!

Thank you, cherished reader, for purchasing my book and taking the time to read it. As a special reward for your decision, I would like to offer a gift of free and discounted books directly to your inbox. All you need to do is fill in the box below with your email address and name to start getting amazing offers in the comfort of your own home. You will never miss an offer because a reminder will be sent to you. Never miss a deal and get great deals without having to leave the house! Subscribe now and start saving!

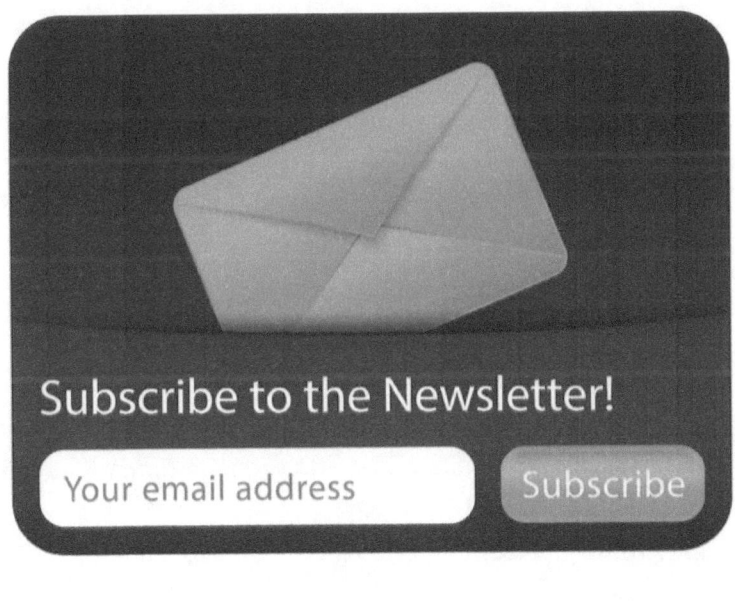

Subscribe to the Newsletter!

Your email address   Subscribe

* * * ★ ★ ★ ★ ★ ★ * * *

Table of Contents

Chapter I: High Fiber Smoothie Recipes

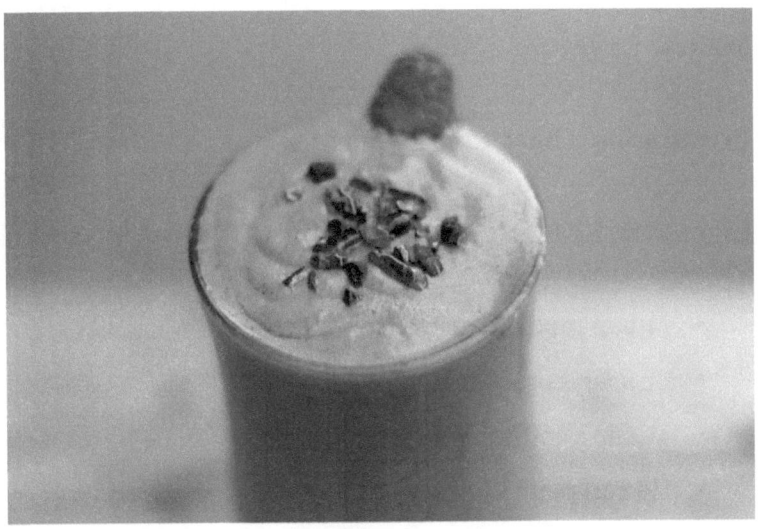

ZZZZZZZZZZZZZZZZZZZZZZZZZZZZZZZZZZZZZZZZZZZZZZZZZZZZZZZZZZ

1) Berry Yogurt Smoothie

This delicious yogurt smoothie is a perfect fiber-rich, on-the-go breakfast alternative.

Makes: 1 to 2

Preparation Time: 15 to 20 minutes

Ingredient List:

- 1 cup mixed berries, frozen
- 1 pear, cored and chopped
- 1 cup vanilla soy milk
- ½ cup plain Greek yogurt

zzzzzzzzzzzzzzzzzzzzzzzzzzzzzzzzzzzzzzzzzzzzzzzzzzzzzzzzzzz

Instructions:

1: Place all ingredients into a blender and blend until smooth.

2: Pour the smoothie into a glass. Consume immediately.

2) Mean Green Smoothie

This green smoothie is filled with vitamins and nutrients, including the much needed fiber.

Makes: 1 to 2

Preparation Time: 15 to 20 minutes

Ingredient List:

- 1 cup green tea, strongly brewed
- ½ avocado, seed removed
- 1 cup baby spinach, fresh
- ½ Tbsp. coconut oil
- ½ to 1 tsp. honey
- 1 cup mango chunks
- Dash of sea salt

zzzzzzzzzzzzzzzzzzzzzzzzzzzzzzzzzzzzzzzzzzzzzzzzzzzzzzzzz

Instructions:

1: Place all the ingredients into a blender.

2: Blend the ingredients until smooth.

3: Transfer the green smoothie into a tall glass and enjoy.

3) Raspberry Smoothie

Raspberry are well known for their high fiber content, so it's only responsible to use them for a fiber rich smoothie.

Makes: 1 to 2

Preparation Time: 15 minutes

Ingredient List:

- 2 cups raspberries, frozen
- ½ cup lemon juice, freshly squeezed
- ½ cup baby spinach, fresh
- ½ cup lime juice, freshly squeezed

zzzzzzzzzzzzzzzzzzzzzzzzzzzzzzzzzzzzzzzzzzzzzzzzzzzzzzzz

Instructions:

1: Place all 4 ingredients into a blender.

2: Blend the ingredients together until smooth.

3: Transfer the smoothie into a glass and enjoy while still cold.

4) Green Tea Weight Loss Smoothie

This fiber-rich smoothie can help aid in fat loss.

Makes: 1 to 2

Preparation Time: 15 to 20 minutes

Ingredient List:

- ¾ cup green tea, strongly brewed
- 2 tsp. agave nectar
- 2 ½ tsp. lemon juice
- 1/8 tsp. cayenne pepper
- 2 Tbsp. plain Greek yogurt
- 1 pear, cored and diced
- 6 ice cubes

zzzzzzzzzzzzzzzzzzzzzzzzzzzzzzzzzzzzzzzzzzzzzzzzzzzzzzzzzzzzzzzz

Instructions:

1: Place all ingredients into a blender.

2: Blend the ingredients until smooth.

3: Pour the smoothie into a glass and enjoy.

5) Pineapple Smoothie Freeze

To improve the healthiness of this fiber rich smoothie, make sure to use juice that is either low in sugar or sugar free.

Makes: 1

Preparation Time: 15 to 20 minutes

Ingredient List:

- 1 cup pineapple chunks, frozen
- 1 pear, cored and chopped
- 1 cup kale, fresh
- 1 cup pineapple juice
- ½ cup ice

zzzzzzzzzzzzzzzzzzzzzzzzzzzzzzzzzzzzzzzzzzzzzzzzzzzzzzzzzz

Instructions:

1: Place all ingredients into a blender.

2: Blend until the mixture is smooth.

3: Pour the smoothie into a tall glass and enjoy as soon as possible.

Chapter II: High Fiber Breakfast Recipes

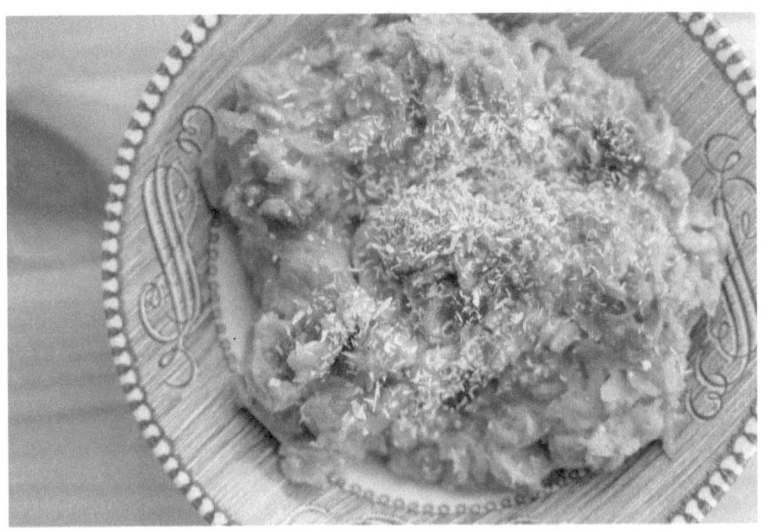

ZZZZZZZZZZZZZZZZZZZZZZZZZZZZZZZZZZZZZZZZZZZZZZZZZZZZZZZZZZ

6) Breakfast Granola

This breakfast granola is a great make-a-head meal that you can grab and eat while you run out the door. It's also high in fiber, making it beneficial for a healthy lifestyle.

Makes: 10

Preparation Time: 1 hour 45 minutes

Ingredient List:

- 1 ¼ cups dates, pitted and diced
- 2 bananas, peeled and diced
- ¼ cup hot water
- ¼ cup brown sugar, packed
- 1 tsp. cinnamon
- 1 Tbsp. vanilla
- 8 ounces slivered almonds, blanched
- 8 cups oats, quick cooking
- 8 ounces dried fruit, mixed

zzzzzzzzzzzzzzzzzzzzzzzzzzzzzzzzzzzzzzzzzzzzzzzzzzzzzzzzzz

Instructions:

1: Turn the oven to 250-degrees and let preheat.

2: In a food processor, puree the dates and bananas. Pour in the hot water, cinnamon, brown sugar and vanilla. Mix until well blended.

3: Transfer the mixture from 2 into a mixing bowl. Place the oats in the mixture and stir.

4: Spread the mixture into a single layer on a cookie sheet. Place in the preheated oven and bake for about 1 ½ hour. Make sure to stir frequently during the baking process. Remove from the oven.

5: Let the baked granola cool before mixing the nuts and dried fruits in.

7) Chia Multigrain Waffles

Waffles are a breakfast staple and these multigrain waffles are filled with fiber to support a healthy diet.

Makes: 8

Preparation Time: 30 to 35 minutes

Ingredient List:

- ½ cup applesauce, unsweetened
- 1 ¾ cups almond milk
- 1 large egg, slightly beaten
- 1 tsp. vanilla
- 2 Tbsp. chia seeds
- ½ cup rolled oats
- 1 ¼ cups flour, whole wheat
- ¼ cup flaxseed meal
- 2 tsp. granulated sugar
- 4 tsp. baking powder
- ¼ tsp. salt

zzzzzzzzzzzzzzzzzzzzzzzzzzzzzzzzzzzzzzzzzzzzzzzzzzzzzzzzzzzzz

Instructions:

1: Turn the waffle iron on and let preheat. Spray the waffle iron with cooking spray.

2: Combine the applesauce, chia seeds, almond milk, egg and vanilla together. Let the mixture sit for about 2 minutes to let the chia seeds thicken the batter.

3: Add the flour, baking powder, salt, sugar. Oats and flaxseed to the applesauce mixture. Mix until just combined.

4: Transfer about ½ cup of the batter into the waffle iron. Cook for about 5 minutes or until the waffles are golden in color and crispy.

5: Continue cooking the waffles in the same manner as above until no batter is left.

6: Serve the waffles warm with your favorite topping, such as syrup.

8) Buckwheat Flapjacks with Blackberries

This flapjack recipe has a double helping of fiber with the buckwheat and the blackberries, the seeds of the fruit is high in fiber.

Makes: 4

Preparation Time: 15 to 20 minutes

Ingredient List:

- ½ cup buckwheat flour
- 1 cup all-purpose flour
- ½ tsp. baking soda
- 1 ½ tsp. baking powder
- 3 Tbsp. granulated sugar
- ½ tsp. salt
- 3 Tbsp. butter, melted
- 2 large eggs
- 1 ½ cup buttermilk
- 1 cup fresh or frozen blackberries

zzzzzzzzzzzzzzzzzzzzzzzzzzzzzzzzzzzzzzzzzzzzzzzzzzzzzzzzzzzzz

Instructions:

1: Mix the two flours together in a large bowl. Add the baking powder, salt, sugar and baking soda and stir until well mixed.

2: In a separate smaller mixing bowl, combine the melted buttermilk, eggs and melted butter together.

3: Carefully pour the milk mixture into the flower mixture and stir until mixed. Keep in mind that there should be lumps in the mixture.

4: Scoop about 1/3 cup of the batter out of the bowl and onto hot, buttered griddle. Sprinkle the blackberries directly on top. Let the pancake cook until bubbles start to form on top. Flip the pancake over and cook the other side for about a minute. Cook the remaining batter in the same manner.

5: Serve the pancakes while warm with your favorite topping, such as maple syrup.

9) Baked Hot Fruit

This delicious breakfast meal is high in fiber and will satisfy that sweet tooth in a relatively healthy manner.

Makes: 8

Preparation Time: 1 hour 45 minutes

Ingredient List:

- 1/3 cup raisins
- 8 ounces apricots, dried
- 8 ounces prunes, pitted
- 1 16-ounce can cherry pie filling
- 1 15-ounce can pineapple chunks, not drained
- 1 cup water
- ¼ cup dry sherry
- 1/3 cup slivered almonds, blanched

ZZZZZZZZZZZZZZZZZZZZZZZZZZZZZZZZZZZZZZZZZZZZZZZZZZZZZZZZZZZZ

Instructions:

1: Turn the oven to 350-degrees and let preheat.

2: Mix the dried apricots, prunes, pineapple and raisins together in a baking dish.

3: In a mixing bowl, combine the water, sherry and cherry pie filling. Pour this mixture over top the ingredients in the baking dish.

4: Place the cover on the baking dish and place in the oven. Bake for about 1 ½ hours. Serve while still warm.

10) Oatmeal

Oatmeal is a belly-filling breakfast that is also high in fiber. Oatmeal is a wonderful meal for anytime of the day.

Makes: 4

Preparation Time: 20 to 25 minutes

Ingredient List:

- 1 cup rolled oats
- 2 cups water
- ½ cup currants, dried
- ¼ tsp. salt
- 1 tsp. ground cinnamon
- 1 cup almond milk
- 4 tsp. honey
- 2 Tbsp. cream

ZZZZZZZZZZZZZZZZZZZZZZZZZZZZZZZZZZZZZZZZZZZZZZZZZZZZZZZZZZZZZ

Instructions:

1: Pour the water in a pot and bring to a boil. Place the oats in the boiling water and stir. Add the salt and stir once again before turning the heat down on low and let simmer for about 5 minutes.

2: Add the currants and stir. Let simmer for about 10 minutes.

3: Remove the oats from heat. Divide the oatmeal between 4 bowls.

4: Sprinkle the cinnamon (about ¼ tsp.) over each oatmeal-filled bowls. Drizzle the honey (about a tsp.) over top each bowl.

5: In a pitcher, mix the almond milk and cream. Serve this mixture on the side of the oatmeal.

Chapter III: High Fiber Lunch Recipes

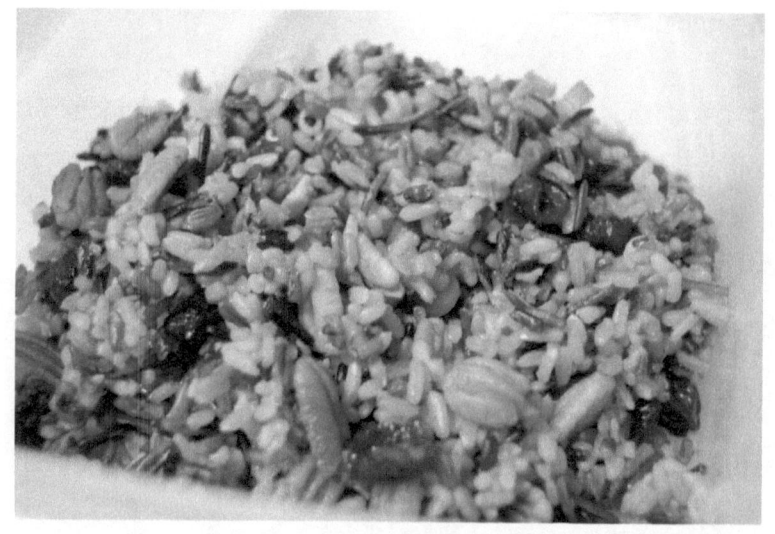

ZZZZZZZZZZZZZZZZZZZZZZZZZZZZZZZZZZZZZZZZZZZZZZZZZZZZZZZZZ

11) Harvest Stew

This hearty stew is a perfect dish for cool days and filled with fiber.

Makes: 6

Preparation Time: 1 hour 30 minutes

Ingredient List:

- 1 pound beef stew cubes
- 2 Tbsp. oil, olive or vegetable
- ¼ cup all-purpose flour
- ¾ cup onions, diced
- ½ cup celery, diced
- ½ cup carrots, sliced
- 6 garlic cloves, peeled
- 1 leek, diced
- 1 potato, skinned and diced
- 2 cups zucchini, diced
- 2 tomatoes, chopped
- 3 turnips, diced
- 3 sprigs thyme
- 1 bay leaf
- 2 Tbsp. Worcestershire sauce
- 4 cups beef broth
- Salt, to taste
- Black pepper, to taste

ZZZZZZZZZZZZZZZZZZZZZZZZZZZZZZZZZZZZZZZZZZZZZZZZZZZZZZZZZZZ

Instructions:

1: Cook the beef in the oil until brown. Stir in the flour until it evenly coats the browned beef.

2: Add the celery, onions, carrots, zucchini, garlic, leek, potato, tomatoes, turnips, beef broth, thyme sprigs and bay leaf. Stir until well mixed.

3: Bring the mixture to a boil before turning the heat down and allowing to simmer for about an hour.

4: Scoop out the thyme sprigs and bay leaf, and discard.

5: Stir in the Worcestershire. Add salt and pepper to taste. Serve the stew while still hot.

12) Wild Rice Salad

Despite its name, wild rice is actually more of a grass then grain. But it is high in fiber none the less.

Makes: 4

Preparation Time: 1 hour 20 minutes

Ingredient List:

- 2 cups wild rice, cooked and warm
- 1 Tbsp. shallots, minced
- ¼ cup yellow bell pepper, diced
- ½ cup walnuts, chopped
- ¼ cup cranberries, dried
- 2 Tbsp. vinegar, balsamic
- 1 Tbsp. walnut oil
- Salt, to taste
- Ground black pepper, to taste

zzzzzzzzzzzzzzzzzzzzzzzzzzzzzzzzzzzzzzzzzzzzzzzzzzzzz

Instructions:

1: Place the cooked and warm wild rice in a large bowl.

2: Add the bell pepper, shallots, cranberries, walnuts, balsamic vinegar, walnut oil, salt and pepper.

3: Toss all the ingredients together until well combined.

4: Cover the bowl and let chill in the fridge for about an hour.

5: Divide the salad between 4 serving bowls and enjoy.

13) Sweet Potato Chicken Soup

This yummy soup recipe is filled with fiber and perfect for those cool and crisp fall and winter afternoons.

Makes: 4

Preparation Time: 60 minutes to 65 minutes

Ingredient List:

- 4 sweet potatoes, peeled and diced
- 1 purple onion, diced
- 1 green onion, chopped
- 2 Tbsp. olive oil
- 2 garlic cloves, minced
- 4 cups chicken broth
- 1 tsp. cinnamon
- 1 tsp. garlic powder
- 1 tsp. paprika
- 4 chicken thighs, cooked, skinned and deboned
- Salt, to taste
- Black pepper, to taste

ZZZZZZZZZZZZZZZZZZZZZZZZZZZZZZZZZZZZZZZZZZZZZZZZZZZZZZ

Instructions:

1: Place the olive oil in a skillet. Heat the oil over medium heat.

2: Add the diced purple onion into the skillet and sauté for about 3 minutes.

3: Add the minced garlic, green onions, paprika and garlic powder and sauté for an additional 2 minutes.

4: Transfer the sautéed ingredients into a large pot. Stir in the diced sweet potato, chicken broth and cinnamon. Turn the heat on high and bring the mixture to a boil. Reduce the heat and let simmer for about ½ hour.

5: Remove the pot from the stove and let cool. Pour the mixture into a blender or food processor and puree. Transfer the mixture back into the pot.

6: Add the meat and stir. Season with salt and black pepper to taste. Let the soup simmer for about 10 minutes. Serve while warm.

14) Cashew and Egg Salad Sandwiches

The added cashews give this egg salad sandwich recipe an extra kick of fiber.

Makes: 2

Preparation Time: 20 minutes

Ingredient List:

- 3 eggs, hard-boiled
- 1 Tbsp. green onions, chopped
- 2 Tbsp. celery, diced
- 1 Tbsp. yogurt, plain
- ¼ cup mayonnaise
- 2 tsp. mustard, Dijon
- 2 tsp. honey
- ¼ cup toasted cashews, chopped
- ¼ tsp. curry powder
- Salt, to taste
- Black pepper, to taste
- 4 leaves green lettuce
- 4 slices bread, multigrain

zzzzzzzzzzzzzzzzzzzzzzzzzzzzzzzzzzzzzzzzzzzzzzzzzzzzzzzz

Instructions:

1: Remove the shells from the hard-boiled eggs. Discard the shells and crumble the eggs. Mix the eggs, green onions and celery together until well distributed.

2: Stir in the yogurt, mayonnaise, honey, mustard and curry powder. Season the mixture to taste with salt and black pepper.

3: Fold the cashews into the egg mixture.

4: Make the sandwiches by spreading the egg salad mixture onto a slice of multigrain bread. Lay a piece of lettuce on top and then position another slice of bread on top.

15) High-Fiber Chili

This delicious chili recipe is high in fiber and takes only 30 or so minutes to make.

Makes: 4

Preparation Time: 30 minutes

Ingredient List:

- 1 pound ground turkey or beef
- 18-ounce can black beans
- 18-ounce can kernel corn
- ½ red onion, diced
- 1 Tbsp. chili powder
- 14-ounce can tomato sauce
- 14-ounce can beef broth
- 1 Tbsp. olive oil
- Shredded cheddar cheese
- Salt, to taste

zzzzzzzzzzzzzzzzzzzzzzzzzzzzzzzzzzzzzzzzzzzzzzzzzzzzzzz

Instructions:

1: Heat the oil in a large cast iron skillet. Add the diced red onion and sauté for about 5 minutes.

2: Add the ground turkey or beef. Use a spatula to crumble the cooking meat. Stir in the chili powder. Continue to cook until the meat has browned. Drain the grease from the meat.

3: Stir in the tomato sauce, beans, corn and broth. Let the mixture start to boil before reducing the heat. Let the mixture simmer for about 10 minutes.

4: Divide the chili between the serving bowls. Sprinkle some cheddar cheese on top before serving.

Chapter IV: High Fiber Dinner Recipes

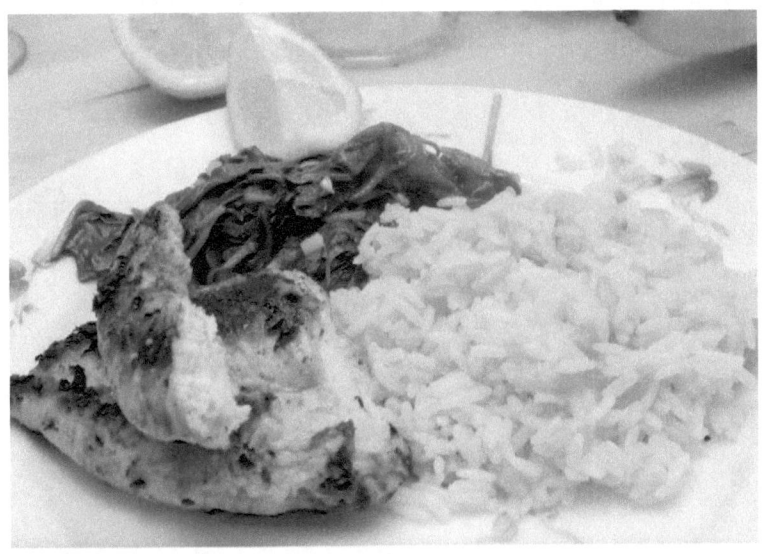

zzzzzzzzzzzzzzzzzzzzzzzzzzzzzzzzzzzzzzzzzzzzzzzzzzzzzzzzzzzz

16) High Fiber Moroccan Chicken

Get a spicy and delicious chicken meal that is also high in fiber with this traditional Moroccan dish.

Makes: 4

Preparation Time: 60 to 65 minutes

Ingredient List:

- 1 pound chicken breast, boneless and skinless
- 1 onion, chopped
- 2 tsp. salt
- 2 carrots, sliced
- 2 garlic cloves, minced
- 2 celery stalks, sliced
- ½ tsp. paprika
- 1 Tbsp. ginger root, minced
- ½ tsp. oregano
- ¾ tsp. cumin
- ¼ tsp. turmeric
- ¼ tsp. cayenne pepper
- 1 ½ cups chicken broth
- 1 cup chickpeas, drained
- 1 cup tomatoes, crushed
- 1 Tbsp. lemon juice
- 1 zucchini, diced

ZZZZZZZZZZZZZZZZZZZZZZZZZZZZZZZZZZZZZZZZZZZZZZZZZZZZZZZZ

Instructions:

1: Season the chicken breasts with salt. Place the seasoned chicken in a large skillet and cook on medium heat. You want the chicken to be cooked almost through. Remove the chicken and set to the side for the moment.

2: In the same pan that you cooked the chicken in, sauté the carrots, garlic, celery and onion until tender. Let cook for about a minute.

3: Add the broth and tomatoes and stir. Transfer the cooked chicken back into the pan. Turn the heat down to low and let the mixture simmer for about 10 minutes.

4: Stir in the zucchini and chickpeas. Turn the heat up a bit and bring to a simmer. Cover the pan and continue to simmer for about 15 minutes.

5: Stir in the lemon juice. Serve with a side of your favorite vegetables.

17) Turkey and Sweet Potato Meatloaf

This delicious meatloaf recipe perfectly blends the flavors of sweet potato and turkey while giving you a fiber boost.

Makes: 4

Preparation Time: 1 hour 30 minutes

Ingredient List:

- 1 pound turkey, ground
- 1 sweet potato, peeled and diced
- 1 large egg
- 2 garlic cloves, minced
- 1 sweet onion, chopped finely
- ¼ cup ketchup
- ¼ cup honey barbecue sauce
- 2 Tbsp. Dijon mustard
- 1 Tbsp. salt
- 1 Tbsp. ground black pepper
- 2 slices whole wheat bread, crumbled

zzzzzzzzzzzzzzzzzzzzzzzzzzzzzzzzzzzzzzzzzzzzzzzzzzzzzzzz

Instructions:

1: Preheat your oven to 350-degrees. Grease the bottom of a 2-quart baking dish. Set to the side for the moment.

2: Place a pot of salted water on the stove and bring to a boil. Carefully submerge the sweet potato into the boiling water and let cook for about 10 minutes or until the potato is tender. Drain the water from the sweet potato.

3: Transfer the tender sweet potato into a small mixing bowl. Mash the sweet potato until smooth.

4: In a large mixing bowl, combined the turkey, sweet onion, egg, garlic, ketchup, barbecue sauce, mustard and crumbled bread together. Add the salt and pepper and stir.

5: Transfer the mashed sweet potato into the turkey mixture. Use your hands to knead the ingredients until well combined.

6: Using your hands, form the mixture into a meatloaf shape. Place the meatloaf in the prepared baking dish.

7: Bake the meatloaf in the preheated oven for about an hour. When cooked through, remove the meatloaf from the oven and slice into loafs.

8: Serve the meatloaf while still warm with your favorite side dish, such as vegetables or pasta.

18) Baked Tilapia

This delicious fish recipe is filled with fiber thanks to the added ingredient Fiber One cereal.

Makes: 2

Preparation Time: 25 to 30 minutes

Ingredient List:

- 1 pound tilapia
- 1 cup Fiber One cereal
- Salt, to taste
- Ground black pepper, to taste
- 1 Tbsp. canola oil
- ¼ cup milk
- 1/3 cup Greek yogurt
- 1 tsp. Dijon mustard
- 1 tsp. horseradish
- 1 onion, chopped

zzzzzzzzzzzzzzzzzzzzzzzzzzzzzzzzzzzzzzzzzzzzzzzzzzzzzzzzz

Instructions:

1: Preheat an oven to 400-degrees. Prepare a baking sheet by spraying the bottom with cooking spray.

2: Fill a plastic Ziplock bag with the cereal. Use a rolling pin to crush the cereal into crumbs.

3: In a shallow bowl, mix the milk, oil, yogurt, basil, horseradish, onion and mustard together.

4: Coat the fish in the milk mixture before placing it in the cereal filled bag and shaking gently until it is completely covered on all sides.

5: Place the coated fish on the prepared baking sheet. Place the baking sheet in the oven and bake for about 15 minutes.

6: Serve the fish with a side of your favorite vegetables.

19) Pork with Black Bean and Peach Salsa

This high-in-fiber dinner has an unusual yet tasty salsa made from black bean and peach.

Makes: 4

Preparation Time: 35 to 45 minutes

Ingredient List:

- 1 pound pork tenderloin, diced
- Salt, to taste
- Ground black pepper, to taste
- 1 Tbsp. olive oil
- ¼ cup cornmeal
- ¼ cup beer
- ½ 15-ounce can black beans, drained with the liquid reserved
- 1 15-ounce can sliced peaches, drained
- 1 cup salsa
- 1 Tbsp. cilantro, chopped

zzzzzzzzzzzzzzzzzzzzzzzzzzzzzzzzzzzzzzzzzzzzzzzzzzzzzzzzzzz

Instructions:

1: Season the pork with pepper and salt. Fill a large Ziploc bag with the cornmeal. Add the seasoned pork and shake the bag until the pork is thoroughly coated.

2: Place the oil in a skillet and heat over medium high. Cook the pork in the skillet and let sauté for about 10 minutes. Reduce the heat to medium.

3: Gradually pour in the beer, peaches, salsa and beans with two Tbsp. of the reserved liquid. Stir the mixture well.

4: Let the mixture simmer for about 20 minutes before stirring in the cilantro. Serve while still warm.

20) Black-Eye Pea Gumbo

This delicious Cajun gumbo is perfect for filling bellies and giving you a healthy dose of fiber.

Makes: 8

Preparation Time: 60 to 75 minutes

Ingredient List:

- 1 Tbsp. oil, vegetable or olive
- 1 green bell pepper, chopped
- 1 onion, chopped
- 5 celery stalks, chopped
- 1 cup brown rice, uncooked
- 2 cups chicken broth
- 4 15-ounce cans black-eye peas, undrained
- 1 14.5-ounce can diced tomatoes
- 1 10-ounce can green chilies and diced tomatoes
- 2 garlic cloves, chopped finely

zzzzzzzzzzzzzzzzzzzzzzzzzzzzzzzzzzzzzzzzzzzzzzzzzzzzzzzzzzzz

Instructions:

1: Place the oil in a large pan. Set the pan on the stove and heat over medium heat.

2: Add the celery, onion and pepper. Sauté until tender.

3: Stir in the chicken broth, rice, diced tomatoes and chilies, diced tomatoes and black-eye peas with its liquid. Add the garlic and stir.

4: Let the mixture being to boil before reducing heat and letting simmer for about 45 minutes. If the soup is too thick, add a bit of water to thin it.

5: Serve the gumbo while still warm.

Chapter V: High Fiber Snack and Dessert Recipes

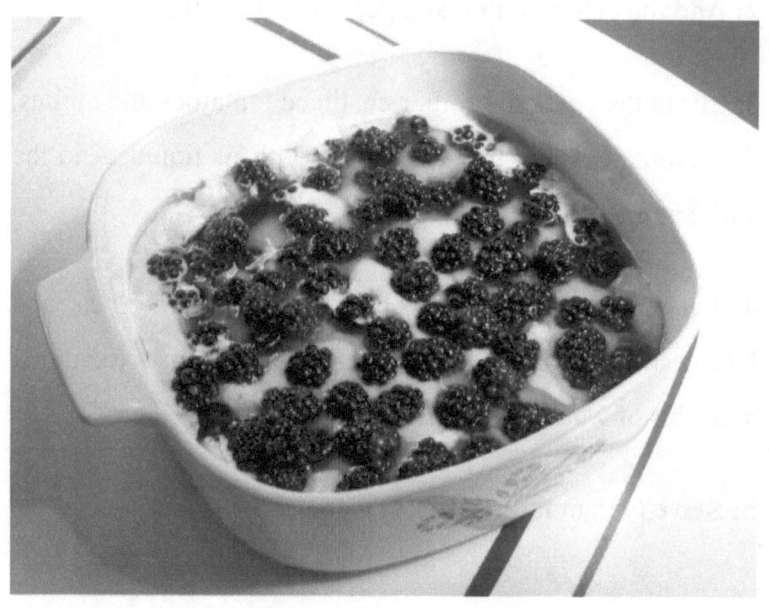

ZZZZZZZZZZZZZZZZZZZZZZZZZZZZZZZZZZZZZZZZZZZZZZZZZZZZZZZZZZZZZZZ

21) Almond Macaroons

It's the addition of applesauce, coconut and candied orange peel that gives these macaroons a boost of fiber.

Makes: 12

Preparation Time: 30 to 40 minutes

Ingredient List:

- 2 egg whites
- ¼ cup applesauce
- ¼ cup granulated sugar
- 1 ¼ cups shredded coconut
- ¾ cup almonds, ground
- ¼ cup candied orange peel, chopped
- 2 Tbsp. flour, all-purpose

ZZZZZZZZZZZZZZZZZZZZZZZZZZZZZZZZZZZZZZZZZZZZZZZZZZZZZZ

Instructions:

1: Preheat the oven to 350-degrees. Prepare a baking pan by lining it with parchment paper.

2: Place the eggs whites and sugar in a mixing bowl. Whip the two ingredients together until frothy.

3: Add the remaining ingredients into the egg/sugar mixture and stir until well combined.

4: Roll the dough into walnut-sized balls. Set the dough balls on to the prepared baking pan. Place the pan in the oven and bake for about 20 minutes.

5: Remove the pan from the oven and let the cookies cool.

22) To-Go Oat Cakes

These fiber packed snacks are like a bowl of oatmeal packed into a to-go cake-like form.

Makes: 8

Preparation Time: 35 to 40 minutes

Ingredient List:

- 2 cups flour, all-purpose
- 3 cups rolled oats
- 1 egg white
- ¼ tsp. baking powder
- ½ cup granulated sugar
- ½ cup plain yogurt
- ½ cup honey
- ½ cup dried apricots, chopped
- ½ tsp. vanilla

zzzzzzzzzzzzzzzzzzzzzzzzzzzzzzzzzzzzzzzzzzzzzzzzzzzzzzzzzz

Instructions:

1: Preheat the oven to 325-degrees. Prepare a baking sheet by lining it with parchment paper. Set to the side for the moment.

2: Add the oats to a food processor and pulse about 10 times. Add the baking soda and flour, and pulse a few more times until mixed.

3: In a mixing bowl, whisk the egg white until it's frothy. Add the honey, sugar, vanilla and yogurt. Mix until well combined.

4: Stir in the pulsed mixture and apricots until well mixed.

5: Roll the dough into 8 equally shaped balls. Flatten the balls into thick patties.

6: Place the patties onto the prepared baking sheet from 1. Bake the patties for about 20 minutes.

7: Remove the patties from the oven and let cool in the fridge.

23) Blackberry Cobbler

Not only is this cobbler delicious, it's also versatile! Don't have blackberries? No problem, you can use cherries, raspberries or blueberries! It's the whole wheat biscuits that gives this recipe the extra fiber.

Makes: 8

Preparation Time: 1 hour 25 minutes

Whole-Wheat Biscuit Ingredient List:

- 1 ½ cups whole-wheat flour
- 1 ½ cups all-purpose flour
- 1 ½ tsp. salt
- 4 ½ tsp. baking powder
- 1 Tbsp. granulated sugar
- 6 Tbsp. butter, cold
- 1 ¾ cups buttermilk

Filling Ingredient List:

- 8 cups blackberries
- ¾ cups granulated sugar
- ¼ cup all-purpose flour
- ¼ cup cream

zzzzzzzzzzzzzzzzzzzzzzzzzzzzzzzzzzzzzzzzzzzzzzzzzzzzzzzzzzzz

Instructions:

1: Make the biscuits by preheating the oven to 350-degrees.

2: Mix the two flours, salt, baking powder and sugar together. Cut the butter into small cubes and mix it into the dry ingredients using a pastry cutter. Pour in the buttermilk and mix well with a wooden spoon.

3: Use a rolling pin to roll the dough onto a floured surface. You want the dough to be about an inch thick. Use a 3-inch cookie cutter to cut the dough into circles. Set the circles to the side for the moment.

4: Prepare the filling by mixing the blackberries with the sugar and flour. Transfer the mixture into a 9x11-inch baking dish. Place the dish in the preheated oven and bake for about 25 minutes.

5: Remove the baking dish from oven. Place the uncooked dough circles directly on top of the filling.

6: Use a pastry brush to brush the tops of the dough circles with cream. Return the baking dish to the oven and bake for an additional 25 minutes.

7: Serve the cobbler while warm with a side of vanilla ice cream if so desired.

24) Energy Balls

If you want a quick snack that isn't lacking in taste or fiber, gives these energy balls a go.

Makes: 12

Preparation Time: 40 to 50 minutes

Ingredient List:

- ½ cup peanut butter, creamy
- ½ cup honey
- 1 cup quick-cook rolled oats, uncooked
- 1 cup nonfat dry milk
- 2 cups corn flakes cereal, crushed
- ½ cup raisins

zzzzzzzzzzzzzzzzzzzzzzzzzzzzzzzzzzzzzzzzzzzzzzzzzzzzzzzz

Instructions:

1: Combine the peanut butter and honey together until smooth.

2: Stir in the oats, dry milk and raisins until well combined.

3: Using your hands, roll the mixture into bite-sized balls.

4: Roll the bite-sized balls into the crushed cereal until it is coated on all sides.

5: Place the balls on a cookie sheet. Cover and let chill in the fridge until firm.

25) Chocolate Chip and Apricot Squares

These yummy cookies are filled with fiber, vitamins and protein so you don't have to feel bad about enjoying these treats.

Makes: 18

Preparation Time: 35 to 40 minutes

Ingredient List:

- 1 cup butter, softened
- ¾ cup granulated sugar
- ¾ cup brown sugar, packed
- 2 eggs, large
- 1 tsp. vanilla
- ½ tsp. salt
- 2 ¼ cups flour, all-purpose
- 1 tsp. baking soda
- 1 cup dried apricots, chopped
- 1 cup chocolate chips
- 1 cup cashews, chopped
- 2 cups granola

ZZZZZZZZZZZZZZZZZZZZZZZZZZZZZZZZZZZZZZZZZZZZZZZZZZZZZZZ

Instructions:

1: Preheat the oven to 375-degrees. Prepare a 9x13-inch baking pan by lining the bottom with foil. Set to the side for the moment.

2: In a large mixing bowl, cream the sugar, brown sugar and butter together until the mixture is fluffy.

3: Stir in the vanilla extract and eggs. Continue mixing until well combined.

4: In a small mixing bowl, shift together the flour, baking soda and salt. Gradually stir this mixture into the sugar mixture.

5: Fold in the apricots, chocolate chips, cashews and granola.

6: Press the dough into the prepared baking pan from 1. Place the pan in the oven and bake for about 20 minutes.

7: Remove the pan from the oven and let cool before cutting into squares.

About the Author

A native of Albuquerque, New Mexico, Sophia Freeman found her calling in the culinary arts when she enrolled at the Sante Fe School of Cooking. Freeman decided to take a year after graduation and travel around Europe, sampling the cuisine from small bistros and family owned restaurants from Italy to Portugal. Her bubbly personality and inquisitive nature made her popular with the locals in the villages and when she finished her trip and came home, she had made friends for life in the places she had visited. She also came home with a deeper understanding of European cuisine.

Freeman went to work at one of Albuquerque's 5-star restaurants as a sous-chef and soon worked her way up to head chef. The restaurant began to feature Freeman's original dishes as specials on the menu and soon after, she began to write e-books with her recipes. Sophia's dishes mix local flavours with European inspiration making them irresistible to the diners in her restaurant and the online community.

Freeman's experience in Europe didn't just teach her new ways of cooking, but also unique methods of presentation. Using rich sauces, crisp vegetables and meat cooked to perfection, she creates a stunning display as well as a delectable dish. She has won many local awards for her cuisine and she continues to delight her diners with her culinary masterpieces.

Author's Afterthoughts

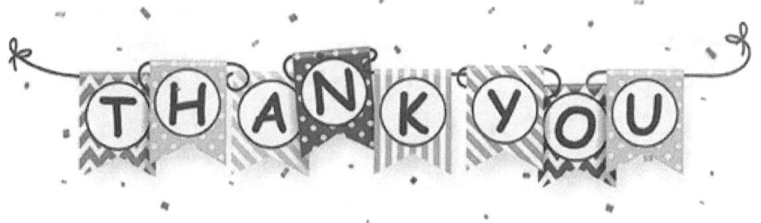

I want to convey my big thanks to all of my readers who have taken the time to read my book. Readers like you make my work so rewarding and I cherish each and every one of you.

Grateful cannot describe how I feel when I know that someone has chosen my work over all of the choices available online. I hope you enjoyed the book as much as I enjoyed writing it.

Feedback from my readers is how I grow and learn as a chef and an author. Please take the time to let me know your thoughts by leaving a review on Amazon so I and your fellow readers can learn from your experience.

My deepest thanks,

Sophia Freeman

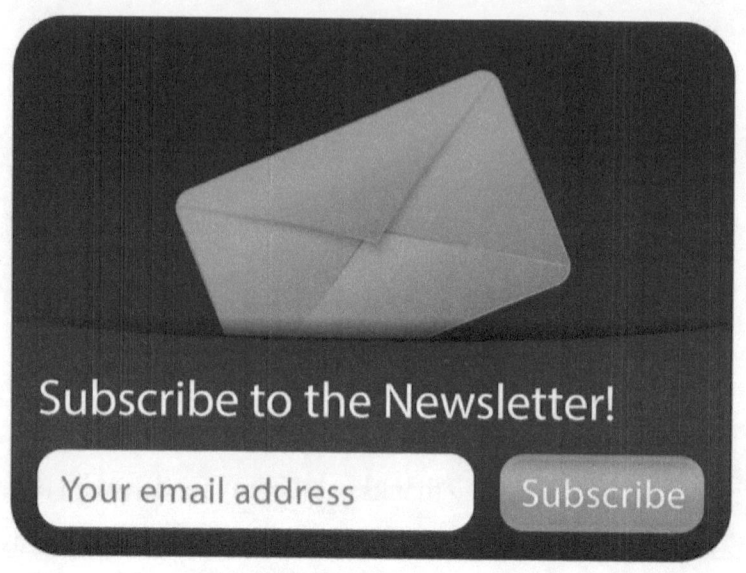

https://sophia.subscribemenow.com/